Intermittent Fasting

Ultimate Guide for Health and Weight Loss

James Statton

Table of Contents

Introduction

Obesity is the leading cause of chronic diseases like diabetes. It is caused by the accumulation of fat in the body. The body needs energy to perform various activities. This energy is normally obtained from the carbs that we eat. The excess of these are stored in the body in the form of fat. This normally leads to a person becoming overweight.

During intermittent fasting, the body will not find food to process and use as the source of energy. In such a case, it turns to burning the fat stored in the body to get energy. This process normally leads to weight loss. This is where fasting becomes important. It makes the body burn the stored fat for energy, aiding in weight loss. This can help one reduce the risk of developing chronic diseases like diabetes. Intermittent fasting is also a natural way of preventing type-2 diabetes. The reason is that it is good for increasing insulin sensitivity, which can help in preventing type-2 diabetes.

Before fasting, one should familiarize themselves with the basics. There are different methods for intermittent fasting, so one must choose the method he likes best. The best method is based on one's goals and lifestyle. There is also a special group of people who should not practice intermittent fasting. You must know whether you are qualified to practice it or not. Intermittent fasting is more concerned about when to eat, not what to eat. During the fasting window, one is not allowed to eat, except ingesting some low-calorie drinks like coffee. During the feeding window, one is allowed to eat the food they need without restriction. For good results, one can combine intermittent fasting with the ketogenic diet. This book is an excellent guide for you on how to practice intermittent fasting. Enjoy reading!

Part 1

12

What Is Intermittent Fasting?

Chapter 1- What Is Intermittent Fasting and Why Is It Good for You?

Intermittent fasting refers to an eating pattern in which one cycles between eating periods and fasting periods. Intermittent fasting doesn't state the kind of foods one should eat, but when they should be eaten. There are different methods of intermittent fasting, but they all divide the day or week into fasting and eating periods.

Nearly everybody fasts daily when asleep, and intermittent fasting may involve only extending this fasting to take a longer period of time. This can be done by not eating breakfast, eating the first meal for the day at noon, and by eating the last meat at night such as at 9:00 PM.

Intermittent fasting has helped people accelerate fat loss and lose weight, gain muscle mass, and become healthier. Intermittent fasting was introduced in 1900s as a way of curing disorders like epilepsy and diabetes. However, it is now gaining traction with modern day dieters.

An example of intermittent fasting is the 5:2 program, which involves eating normally for 5 days a week, then following a modified fasting program for 2 days of the week, during which one should eat very little, between 500-600 calories.

Intermittent fasting is an easy and effective way of losing weight, restricting calories and burning fat. It also has metabolic health benefits. Intermittent fasting enhances the function of hormones to improve weight loss.

Higher levels of growth hormone, lowers levels of insulin, and high levels of norepinephrine increase the rate at which the body fat is broken down and the use of the same as a source of energy. A short term fast increases one's rate of metabolism by 3.6 to 14 percent, helping them burn more calories.

A 2014 review done by scientific literature stated that intermittent fasting causes a weight loss of 3 to 8 percent within 3 to 24 weeks, which is a great amount. It was also found that the individuals lost 4 to 7 percent of the circumference of their waist, meaning a lot of belly fat was lost. Belly fat is very harmful as it causes diseases.

Another study has shown that intermittent fasting causes less muscle loss compared to continuous calorie restriction. Considering all the above, intermittent fasting is a great tool for weight loss.

Intermittent fasting has been found to be good in tempering blood pressure and fluid balance. During a fasting state, blood pressure tends to fall, primarily after fasting for one week. This is due to a low intake of salt, as well as detoxification of salt that had previously accumulated, which is excreted via urine. Intake of sodium causes the body to retain water; lower levels of sodium will lead to a better balance of body fluids.

Fasting is good for brain protection. Calorie restriction and fasting prevent the production of free radicals and irritating proteins such as inflammatory cytokines. As the production of these reduces, the production of protective cytokine increases, protecting the brain from the oxidative damage.

Fasting is a good way of moderating appetite. During fasting, the levels of the hormone leptin drop. As you keep on losing weight, the body's response to leptine will increase, making you feel full for longer. This way, your chances of eating healthy foods will increase. Weight loss experts have stated that leptin resistance prevents overweight individuals from losing weight since they will not be signaled by hormones once their stomachs are full.

Fasting is the key to living healthier and longer. Research has shown that animals that are fed on low-calorie foods live longer than other animals. When organisms face challenges such as famine, more resources will be dedicated for survival. This involves finding more ways for survival, which might make you live longer.

With fasting, humans can achieve an improved immune system. Fasting is known to trigger the recycling of white blood cells, which are the cells responsible for the immune system. When the immune cells are recycled, the end result is a highly competent immune system. This is normally achieved by triggering of regeneration of stem cells which become platelets, white blood cells, and red blood cells once you eat.

Research has shown that fasting may increase one's resistance to mental stress. Fasting leads to stable levels of blood sugar and insulin hormone. This also leads to an improved response to mental stress by the brain and protects the brain from any damage related to stress.

Chapter 2- A Brief History of Fasting

Fasting devotees have claimed that it brings spiritual and physical renewal. After the success of the 5:2 fasting program, a wider audience has known the benefits associated with fasting, hence the need for this to be supervised.

Fasting has been in practice for many years in connection to religious ceremonies. It was first observed in Christians, Jews, Confucianists, Hindus, Muslims, Taoists, Jainists and other religions. Buddhism has a great emphasis on moderation of eating, but it observes some fasts.

Traditionally, fasting was one of the rites which were suspended or reduced, leading to a state of quiescence that can be compared to death, or the state preceding birth. In primitive ceremonies, fasting was part of fertility rites. In the fourteenth century, St. Catherine of Siena practiced fasting.

Primitive cultures practiced fasting before going for war. Native North Americans practiced fasting as a rite of avoiding catastrophes like famine.

Fasting plays a key role in major religions to date, other than Zoroastrianism in which it is prohibited. It is associated with penitence and other kinds of self-control. In Judaism, there are several fasting days per annum, including the Day of Atonement and Yom Kippur. Muslims practice fasting during the holy month of Ramadan. Eastern orthodoxy and Roman Catholics practice a 40 day fasting period during Lent, a way of remembering when Jesus was tempted in the desert for 40 days.

Fasting plays a great role in the major religions of the world even today. However, it takes various forms in these different religions. There are rules that govern fasting at different times of the year or particular dates in religious calendars. Fasting is normally done individually or collectively, complete abstinence or limited diet with no oils, animal products, or stimulants.

Fasting is not as old as the humans on earth, but it is highly topical today as a source of humans' self-healing powers, applied successively in treating diabetic disorders and inflammatory joint.

Chapter 3- Myths of Fasting

There are various myths surrounding fasting. People have come to believe such myths as infallible truths. Here are some of the myths associated with fasting:

1. Fasting will slow your metabolism.
    Low calorie diets and fasting are different with various effects on hormones and general physiology. Fasting leads to an increased rate of release of adrenaline, which increases lipolysis (fat burning) and metabolism. It was a good way for our ancestors to get energy to search for food during famine. This has a different effect than eating a low calorie diet, which slows down metabolism leading to weight gain.
    If it is true that fasting reduces metabolism, then our ancestors who went through long periods of fasting would be fat and fatigued, but they were lean and energetic. Note that eating frequently as a way of boosting metabolism is dangerous as it leads to increased storage of fats and a slow metabolism. It is true that athletes eat this

way, but they already have a high metabolism and their goal is to boost it.

2. Fasting breaks down muscles.

Fasting should not be confused with low calorie diets. Individuals who under-nourish themselves with extreme diets and nutrient deficient cleanses coupled with increased exercise will break down their muscle and gain fat.

The human body is made to preserve muscle during fasting, and that's why fasting leads to the release of growth hormone. Human bodies have enough glucose stores in the muscle and the liver which is accessed first during fasting. Once the stored glucose is over, the body turns to the stored fat. Breaking down of muscles to get body energy is the last resort.

Today's professionals are adopting intermittent fasting as a way of retaining lean muscle and burning fat. It is a good strategy for non-athletic types. Some of the reasons as to why individuals break down muscle include lack of sleep, sedentary lifestyle, protein-deficient diets, and chronic stress.

3. Fasting causes hunger and overeating.

Fasting doesn't cause hunger and overeating, but eating does. This is the case with eating modern day foods that are full of sugar and other artificial ingredients that are made to be addictive.

If you rely on the standard diet of today, your hunger is caused by insulin and glucose levels that surge then crash during the day. You don't control your food, but the food controls you. In such a case, you are not recommended to fast. Begin by eating a clean diet. Once your body attains a point of stable insulin levels, you will be prepared through a period of intermittent fasting. If you rely on a poor diet then you try to fast, it will be a torture to you and you may never fast again.

Before beginning to fast, your metabolic machinery and hormones must be prepared to take you through the fast.

4. Fasting will reduce blood glucose making it too low.

Your body is a machine for glucose making and storage. With time, the levels of glucose become stable, and improvements are seen, including a reversal in the insulin resistance conditions such as diabetes.

Hypoglycemia (a condition caused by extremely low blood glucose) is a precaution only for diabetics taking oral pills or insulin for lowering blood glucose. In such a case, you should closely monitor the level of your blood glucose under the watch of a health professional if you need to do fasts.

You may have to begin with short fasting intervals while watching your glucose levels. If the insulin levels show consistent improvement, your physician may taper down insulin-lowering medications or injectable insulin.

The point here is that intermittent fasting leads to stable blood glucose levels and can reverse diabetes.

5. Fasting is hard.

Fasting is natural, and it's encoded into human DNA. However, modern life has made it hard for humans to fast. If you eat your dinner before 8:00 PM, skip breakfast the following day, and have an early lunch at noon, then you will have gone through a 16 hour fast.

Remember that skipping breakfast won't slow down your metabolism. Avoid the studies you have read about an improvement in weight loss for those who eat breakfast. The reason they say this is that some are done under confounding factors while others are sponsored by the breakfast cereal companies. If you eat breakfast and you maintain a healthy body, then there is no need for you to skip it. If you need to lose weight, and you don't feel hungry in the morning, there is no need to force food into your mouth.

When eating, choose foods dense in nutrients and rich in proteins, vegetables, and healthy fats. If fasting becomes tough for you, go to bed earlier than usual, and use the bedtime as the fasting hours. This will also help you generate more growth hormone. If you go to bed late at night, you might munch on food before bedtime, and it will also lead to less production of growth hormone.

Take some occasional times and fast, while determining the impact it has on your health, ability to focus, body composition, and the level of blood glucose.

6. Fasting increases cortisol levels, causing stress.
    Cortisol is the stress hormone responsible for
    maintaining blood pressure and regulating the
    immune system. It is good for breaking down
    protein and glucose. Many people demonize
    this hormone, but it plays a great role in the
    human body. It's responsible for getting you
    out of bed and getting you moving. Individuals
    who experience low levels of cortisol on a
    regular basis suffer from depression. The levels
    of cortisol rise after exercising, and this helps
    in mobilizing body fat. Short term fasting
    doesn't impact the cortisol levels in your body.
    In one of the studies done about this, it was
    found that fasting individuals experienced
    reduced levels of cortisol. You should note that
    fasting will not increase your cortisol levels,
    but it may reduce them.

7. Fasting causes overeating
    You must have heard some people argue that
    fasting doesn't help reduce weight as it will
    lead to overeating once you begin eating. This
    is partly true, but not wholly true. It is true
    that some people may eat too much after
    fasting than what they would eat with no

fasting. However, research has shown that they only eat 500 extra calories. They may seem to be a lot, but considering that people lose 2400 calories while fasting, this leads to a calorie consumption of 1900 in the red.

Intermittent fasting will lead to a reduced level of food consumption while at the same time boosting the rate of metabolism.

It leads to reduced insulin levels while boosting human growth hormone (HGH) to five times its normal amount.

8. Fasting is not good for general health.
   People believe that fasting may harm your body. However, science has shown that this is not true. Numerous studies have shown that intermittent fasting is good for the body. In animal studies, fasting has been found to turn on genes that cause longevity and protect from diseases. Intermittent fasting has been found to reduce inflammation and oxidative stress and cause an improved sensitivity to insulin.

9. Fasting will put you into starvation mode.
   Most people believe this myth is true. They believe that when fasting, the body believes it is starving, shutting down the metabolism as a

way of conserving fats and calories. A long-term weight loss will lead to a reduction in the number of calories that you burn, and it may add up to hundreds of calories that are burned per day. However, remember that this will happen with weight loss despite the weight method that you use. This won't happen more with fasting than with any other diet plan. Research has shown that short term fasting leads to increased rates of metabolism. The reason is that they cause drastic increases in the level of noradrenaline in the blood, telling the fat cells to break down and be ready for use. The metabolism will in turn be stimulated to prepare itself for the incoming calories and fats.

Chapter 4- Advantages of Fasting

Fasting has been found to be very good, especially in curing diabetes. Diabetes is a disease characterized by high blood sugar, which is simply excess blood glucose. This problem is caused by insulin. The work of insulin is to make the body cells take glucose from the blood. For the case of individuals with diabetes, the glucose stays in the blood since the cells don't take it. Part of the cause is that the cells lose their sensitivity to insulin. Another reason is that the pancreas stops making insulin.

With periodic fasting, the pancreas can be made to start producing insulin. During the period of restricted eating, the pancreas is given time to remove and recycle most of its cells. After a person begins to eat again, the new cells begin to release insulin.

Insulin Resistance

After your body gets too much sugar and carbs, it can become resistant to insulin, and this can lead to many chronic disease like type-2 diabetes. Once insulin sends signals to the body cells that fuel is on the way, and the cells in turn respond by getting glucose from the bloodstream, you will get the energy that you need, and you will not store body fat.

In case of insulin resistance, this does not happen. The insulin signals the body that fuel is on the way, but the cells don't respond by receiving the glucose. Sugar will be kept in the bloodstream and after sometime, the body will store it in the form of fat.

The body will also respond to the failure of its cells to respond to insulin. The pancreas will release more insulin to raise the volume on the signal that the body's cells should absorb glucose. In some cases, the cells only need a small amount of insulin to respond. Insulin resistance occurs when the body cells are stubborn and fail to respond well to the insulin signal for a number of reasons.

The pancreas usually tries to counter this by producing more and more insulin. At some point, the pancreas will be fatigued, and you will suffer from insulin deficiency, diabetes, or pre-diabetes. The resultant effect of these occurrences is increased blood glucose and more fat storage.

Most people with insulin resistance are not aware and may go for long periods of time without the energy that their body needs. The following are some of the symptoms that may be attributed to insulin resistance:

- Fatigue
- Dark skin patches (acanthosis nigricans)
- Acne
- Extra weight at the middle
- High fasting blood sugar
- Polycystic ovarian syndrome
- Carb and sugar cravings
- Fatty liver disease
- Skin tags
- Loss of scalp hair in women
- High blood pressure
- Fluid retention and swelling in the ankles
- Trouble concentrating

To avoid these symptoms, keep your body sensitive to insulin. Fasting is one of the ways to achieve this. It has been found to be good in increasing insulin resistance. A research study published in *World Journal of Diabetes* states intermittent fasting in individuals with type-2 diabetes helped them greatly improve symptoms, including glucose levels and body weight. Another study found that intermittent fasting is as good as caloric restrictions in reduction of visceral fat mass, insulin resistance, and fasting insulin. For individuals struggling with insulin sensitivity or pre-diabetes, intermittent fasting is a good way to get things working.

When an individual develops insulin resistance, the body will always try to shove the energy into fat cells, making you feel tired, cold, and lousy. Resistance does not depend on the high levels, but it depends on the persistence of the high levels.

Intermittent fasting is the easiest way for one to fast, and it can help you cure insulin resistance. It requires you to eat all the food that you have wanted to eat during the day within a short period of time. Most people fast for between 12 to 20 hours each day, and it all depends on their goals.

Intermittent fasting will help you to reset your sensitivity to insulin. You may find it hard to skip breakfast or both breakfast and lunch. However, there is a lot that you can do to make it easier for you. Eating a pure fat breakfast, without carbs or proteins, will send a signal to your body that you are not starving, and you will not have screwed up your intermittent fast.

Once the body burns all the available glucose, it will move to burn glycogen, which is the stored glucose. Once the stores have been exhausted, the body will be put into the process of ketosis, which is a process in which ketones are made for energy. Butter coffee, also called bulletproof coffee, helps you fill up without breaking your fast, and its specific fat profile will help you create ketones at a faster rate to maintain a high level of energy making you prevent hunger.

While doing intermittent fasting, we recommend that you get a glucose meter. Then, keep on checking yourself regularly. If you want to try intermittent fasting, get a ketosis and combo glucose meter so as to monitor both. Track how your clothes fit, your weight, your numbers, and keep on checking the way you feel. That way, you will be able to tell when you attain the best version of yourself.

Chapter 5- The Science Behind Intermittent Fasting

Autophagy means "eating oneself." It is the mechanism by which the body gets rid of all the broken down and old cell machinery (proteins, organelles, and cell membranes) when there isn't enough energy for sustaining it. It is an orderly and regulated process for degrading and recycling cellular components.

The process of apoptosis is well known as programmed cell death. The process is good for one to maintain good health. The body cells normally become junky and old with time. They are programmed to die when their useful days are over. That is what apoptosis entails, in which cells are programmed to die after a certain period of time.

The same process is also done at the sub-cellular level. Instead of having to kill the whole cell, you may only need to replace some of its parts. This is the same as when you have an old car. You don't to replace the entire car, but maybe its battery or the tires and continue using the other old parts. That is how the process of *autophagy* happens, in which the sub-cellular organelles are destroyed, and new ones are created to replace them. Old organelles, cellular membranes, and cellular debris may be removed. This is achieved after sending it to lysosome, an organelle with enzymes responsible for degrading proteins.

The main activator of autophagy is nutrient deprivation. Note that the glucagon hormone can be seen to be the opposite of insulin. If insulin goes down, then glucagon goes up. If insulin goes up, glucagon goes down. During fasting, insulin goes down while glucagon goes up. The increase in the glucagon levels leads to autophagy. Fasting is known to be the greatest booster to the process of autophagy.

Autophagy can be seen as a form of cellular cleansing. This marks the substandard and old cellular equipment for destruction. Fasting offers additional benefits rather than simply stimulating autophagy. When autophagy is stimulated, all junky and old cellular parts and proteins are cleared. Fasting is good for stimulating the release of growth hormone, which triggers the body to begin producing some new parts. Fasting is a good way of giving the body a complete renovation. This means that fasting can work miracles in reversing the aging process by removing the old cellular junk then replacing it with new ones.

Intermittent fasting shines in improving hormones with a direct effect on blood sugar, hunger, and metabolism. It is a fact that intermittent fasting reduces insulin resistance, which enhances metabolism and reduces the risk of diabetes. Intermittent fasting has a positive effect on ghrelin, which is a hunger hormone. A change in the release of ghrelin during intermittent fasting improves the levels of dopamine in the brain, which is good for improved cognitive function. Leptin resistance, a hormonal resistance that leads to stubborn weight gain, benefits from intermittent fasting.

Intermittent fasting has an impact on the female hormones estrogen and progesterone. The brain communicates with the ovaries via brain-ovary axis by sending hormones, which can be seen as chemical emails, to the ovaries, stimulating them to release estrogen and progesterone hormones. For general well-being, your HPG should be healthy. It is also essential for one to get pregnant.

Women are a bit more sensitive to intermittent fasting due to kisspeptin. Women have more kisspeptin, which makes them more sensitive to things like fasting. Due to this, women who go through intermittent fasting may throw off their cycle, miss their periods, or feel hormonally unbalanced. This may also affect metabolism and fertility.

The adrenal glands, located on top of the kidneys, are responsible for the secretion of cortisol, the stress hormone. Adrenal fatigue occurs when the brain-adrenal (HPA) balance goes out of whack. Cortisol may then be high when it's supposed to be low, and low when it's supposed to be high, or always stay low or high. This means HPA-axis dysfunction can occur in various ways.

Thyroid hormones have an effect on all the cells of your body. This means if your thyroid doesn't work, nothing in your body will work. There are various causes of issues related to the thyroid hormone. The thyroid hormone disorders respond differently to intermittent fasting. It is recommended that you consult your medical doctor before beginning fasting and he/she will recommend what to do based on your case.

Part 2

How to Fast

Chapter 6- Different IF Methods

Intermittent fasting has gained popularity in recent years. It is known to improve metabolic health, aid weight loss, and even improve one's lifespan. It is a good way for one to loose body fat while maintaining their muscle mass instead of losing both. It helps in improving the amount of triglycerides and cholesterol in both the overweight and those normal weight.

Individuals have adopted different methods for intermittent fasting. These methods have different effects on different people. Individuals are advised to choose the method that will make life easiest for them. If you don't, the method you choose may not be sustainable, and you may not get the results that you want.

Each method has its own guidelines that director the individuals on how long to fast and what they should eat. Note that not everybody should practice intermittent fasting. Individuals with health conditions are advised to consult their doctors before changing their eating routines. Your lifestyle and personal goals should guide you when choosing a method for intermittent fasting. Let us discuss the command methods for intermittent fasting:

Leangains

This method was started by Martain Berkhan, and it is suitable to individuals addicted to the gym for losing body fat and gaining muscle.
With this method, one is expected to fast for 14 (women) to 16 (men) hours, then eat for the remaining 8 to 10 hours of the day. One should not consume any calories during the fasting period. However, you are allowed to consume black coffee, tea, diet soda, calorie-free sweeteners, and sugar-free gum. You can add a splash of milk into your coffee. Most individuals find it a bit easier to fast during the night into the morning with this method. They stop the fasting six hours after waking up. It is a very flexible fasting schedule to anyone regardless of their lifestyle, but it will be good for them to maintain a consistent feeding window. Failure to do this may throw the body hormones out of whack, which might make it hard to stick to the program.
When and what you consume during the eating period will be determined by when you go for a

workout. During the days of workouts, carbs will be of much more importance than fats. During the day of rest, you should eat higher fats. The consumption of proteins should be high each day, but this will be determined by your goals, body fat, gender, age, and levels of activity. Your calorie intake should be composed of whole, unprocessed foods regardless of the kind of program you are following. If you don't have time for a meal, you are allowed to take a meal replacement bar or a protein shake.

Advantages:

This method has an advantage to most people in that the meal frequency is not relevant. You are allowed to eat anytime within the eight-hour feeding window. Due to this, people have broken this period into three meals which is easy for anyone to stick to as we have been programmed to stick to that feeding schedule.

Disadvantages:

It is true that Leangains provides individuals with a lot of flexibility as far as the time to eat is concerned. However, there is a lot of restriction as to what to eat, especially during workouts. The nutrition restrictions and scheduling of meals may make it harder to follow the program.

Eat Stop Eat

This intermittent fasting method was introduced by Brad Pilon and is suitable for healthy eaters in need of an extra boost.

The method involves fasting for 24 hours once or twice every week. During the 24-hour fasting period, one is only allowed to take calorie-free beverages. Once the fasting period is over, one goes back to eating normally. You should act as if you didn't fast. With this program, you can reduce your intake for calories without actually having to limit what you eat. If your goal is to reduce weight or improve your body composition, it would be good for you to combine it with regular workouts to attain success.

Advantages:

Fasting for 24 hours may seem to be a long period, but the program provides a lot of flexibility. At the beginning, you don't have to do an all-or-nothing fast. For the first day, go as long as you can without taking food, then increase this period gradually in the next few days. This will help you give your body time to adjust. The fast should be started on a day you know you are busy and when you are sure you don't have eating obligations.

Also, there are no forbidden foods, no restricting your diet or weighing food, and no counting calories, making the program easier to follow. Note that with this program, you can eat what you want, but not as much as you want.

Disadvantages:

At the start, it may be difficult for some people to go for 24 hours without taking in any calories. Some people have complained of struggling with going for so long without food, complaining of symptoms like fatigue, headache, or getting anxious, although most of these symptoms die with time. Due to the long fasting period, it is easy for one to find themselves bingeing after the fast. It is possible for this to be controlled, but a lot of self-control is needed, which most people don' have.

The Warrior Diet

This intermittent fasting method was introduced by Ori Hofmekler, and it fits the devoted ones or the people good at following rules.

The method involves fasting for 20 hours each day and taking one large meal at night. The method also considers when you eat and what you eat for the one large meal. The philosophy behind the method is feeding the body with the nutrients it needs in line with circadian rhythms and that we are nocturnal eaters programmed to eat at night.

The Warrior Diet's fasting period is more about under-eating. One is allowed to take a few servings of veggies or raw fruit fresh juice and even some servings of protein if needed. This will maximize the flight or fight response by the sympathetic nervous system which boosts energy, promotes alertness, and stimulates burning of fat.

The four-hour eating window is done at night to maximize the ability of parasympathetic nervous system in promoting calmness, recuperating the body, digestion, and relaxation. The body will also be allowed to use the nutrients that were consumed for growth and repair. When you eat during the night, the body will be forced to burn fat and produce hormones. During the four hours, the order in which the various food groups are eaten is of importance. It is recommended that you begin with veggies, then proteins, and lastly fats. Once you have eaten foods from those groups, you can only go for carbs if you're not full.

Advantages:

Most people like this intermittent fasting method because even in the fasting hours, one is allowed to eat snacks, making it easy for one to get through. Many practitioners have also associated this with increased levels of energy and high rate of fat loss.

Disadvantages:

It is true that you are allowed to eat some snacks during the 20-hour fast, but you are restricted on the kind of snacks to eat, which might make it hard to follow. The strict meal plan and schedule may affect social gatherings. It may also be tough for people to eat one meal only at night while following restrictions on what to it for this meal. It is hard for individuals who don't like eating large meals at night.

Fat Loss Forever

This method was introduced by John Romaniello and Dan Go, and it is good for gym goers who enjoy cheat days. If you've not been satisfied by any of the intermittent fasting methods discussed above, this is the best one for you. It takes the best aspects from the three intermittent fasting methods above, that is, Eat Stop Eat, Leangains, and The Warrior Diet, and combines them into one. Fasters also get one cheat day every week which is followed by a fast of 36 hours. The remaining seven-day cycle is divided between the various fasting protocols.
It is recommended that the longest fasts should be done during the busiest days as this will allow the individual to focus on being productive. Training programs accompany the plan to help the participants attain maximum fat loss in the simplest way.

Advantages:

It is known that every individual fasts daily during the hours that they are not eating. However, this is not done in the right way; hence, don't see and enjoy its benefits. This method provides a seven-day fasting schedule for the body to get used to the schedule and reap maximum benefits from the fasts. One also gets a full cheat day, which everyone loves.

Disadvantages:

For individuals who can't handle cheat days in a healthy way, this method won't suit them. The plan is also very specific with the feeding/fasting schedule varying from day to day. This may confuse the practitioners, finding it hard to follow the plan.

UpDayDownDay Diet

This intermittent fasting plan is also known as the *Alternate-Day Diet,* and it was started by James Johnson, M.D. It is good for disciplined dieters who have a specific goal weight.
The method involves eating very little one day then eating normally the next day. During the low-calorie days, you should eat a fifth of the normal calorie

intake. If men take in 2500 calories, women take 2000 calories, they should take 500 and 400 calories respectively during the fasting day.

To adhere to the plan, meal replacement shakes are highly recommended. These are full of essential nutrients, and you can drink them during the entire day instead of having to split them between meals. However, meal replacement shakes are only recommended for the first two weeks of fasting. After that, one should rely on real food during the "real" days. On the next day, one should eat normally. It is recommended that you should keep workouts during these days on the tamer side, or just save sweat sessions for the normal calorie days.

Advantages:

The method is only about weight loss, fitting those in need of shedding some pounds. On average, individuals who cut calories by 20 to 35 percent lose two and half pounds every week.

Disadvantages:

The method is easy for one to follow, but it also easy for individuals to binge during the normal days. That is why it is recommended that individuals should plan their meals ahead on time to avoid bingeing. This way, you will not be caught by a buffet or at the drive-through on a hungry stomach.

5:2 Diet

This is a simple method to follow. It involves eating normally for five days, not worrying about calories. On the other two days of the week, men should restrict their calories to 600 while women to 500 per day.

The fast days may be tough, but you are encouraged to spread the meals as much as possible and eat less calorie foods like veggies, and eat a good amount of these. Veggies are known to be low in calories. Two cups full of salad greens, for example, will provide less than forty calories. You may add other veggies to this, and come up with a low-calorie salad. This will leave you filled up. If you consume high calorie foods, like fatty foods and fried foods, then the calories will add up quickly.

It will be good to pay attention to what you eat, and stick to low calorie foods to avoid the feeling of being deprived. Soups are good for fasting individuals, especially the ones filled with broth as they will make one feel full.

Note that it doesn't matter the days you choose to fast on. During the initial fasting days, ensure you have at least one non-fasting day in between the fasting days. It is true that you can eat whatever you want to eat during the non-fasting days. However, if you binge on bad foods, like junk foods or fatty foods, you may not see the results that you expect. Instead of losing weight, you may end up gaining more. During the off days, we recommend that you eat a clean diet, choosing foods low in calories and you will see the fruits. In the long run, you will reach your health goals.

Those are the intermittent fasting methods that we have. Note that none of them can be said to fit a particular individual. You only have to try them, and choose the best one that fits you. To know this, you have to keep checking how you progress in terms of weight and how you feel. Once you have identified the best method, stick to it, and you will enjoy results from the fasts. Before sticking to one method, ensure you have tried nearly all of them. However, you may also go for recommendations from your friends, relatives, or your medical doctor. If you have a special condition, also consider a medical professional to give you the necessary instructions on what to do.

Chapter 7- Fasting for General Health

Fasting is different from starvation. For individuals fasting for health purposes, it is simply a structured way of eating. In religion, fasting is mostly succeeded by a feasting period. In some fasts, tea, water, coffee, and other fluids are permitted during fasting, but dry fasts go without these.

Most of the studies done about fasting have involved animals, but the practice has been found to be very beneficial to humans. Fasting has been found that it provides mental clarity and sharpens one's mind. The fact is that the majority of the benefits associated with fasting are not directly as a result of fasting but from the reduced intake of calories, better sleep, decreased fat composition, and lower salt intake.

Before beginning to fast, one must know the schedule and nutrition. You should also have realistic goals when fasting. Emotional or unhealthy eating patterns, inadequate sleep, and poor stress management techniques may hinder you from seeing the health benefits of fasting.

While fasting for general health, one should stay hydrated. During the first few days of fasting, say three days, you may experience some mild symptoms as the body tries to adjust to this. Some of these symptoms include hunger, slight headache, irritability ,and disorientation. During the fourth day, you will begin to feel better than you felt when beginning the fast.

There are categories of people that should not fast. These include pregnant women, children, and lactating women. Diabetics should not fast unless authorized to do so by a trusted health professional. They are encouraged to converse with their doctor, then get an informed opinion that is personalized according to the needs and the situation the individual is in before changing their diet and beginning to fast.

The body changes you will notice during fasting will be determined by the length of the continuous fasting period. The body enters a fasting state about eight hours after the last meal when all the nutrients have been absorbed by the gut. The body turns to break down the body fat to get energy, a process known as *metabolism.* This also helps in the preservation of muscles.

When fat is used as a source of energy, weight loss is triggered. This reduces the levels of cholesterol and preserves your muscle.

After some days of fasting, your blood will have higher levels of endorphins, and you will have a general feeling of mental wellbeing.

One is encouraged to eat a balanced diet with plenty of fluid in between fasts. The kidneys are good for regulating the levels of salt and water in the body, but a lot of these are lost through sweating. Proteins are good for muscle building during fasts.

Effects of Fasting on General Health

The following are some of the impacts of fasting on general health:

1. Weight loss

    Instead of getting energy from the food you eat, fasting will make the body turn to stored fat to get energy from them. The effect of this will be a slow loss of weight, which is good for general health. Fasting is a change of lifestyle, making it easy for most people to adhere to for a long time. This means after attaining the weight you have wanted, it will be easy for you to maintain it.

Being overweight is associated with a number of diseases like diabetes and heart attack. With fasting, you will reduce your weight; hence, you will be safe from this.

2. Improved glucose tolerance

For those with diabetes, fasting is a good way to regulate glucose and improve its variability. If you need a natural way of improving insulin sensitivity, intermittent fasting is the best. The reason is that fasting brings a lot of changes in terms of how the body processes glucose. Insulin resistance develops from the accumulation of glucose in tissues that were not made for fat storage. As the body burns stored fat, the accumulation reduces to become smaller, and the muscle cells, as well as cells in other tissues, grow, increasing insulin sensitivity. If you want to not depend on medications anymore, then try intermittent fasting.

3. Boosting metabolism

   Fasting is characterized by going through periods of not eating followed by periods of eating. This can trigger the process of metabolism. It is true that long-term fasts may slow down the process of metabolism, but short term fasts facilitated by intermittent fasting lead to a fast rate of metabolism. Fasting is more effective compared to long-term calorie restriction since the latter can distort your metabolism. With intermittent fasting, you will also maintain your muscles, which is not the case with calorie restriction.

4. Reduced disorders

   Research has shown that intermittent fasting is a good way of reducing and preventing disorders that can lead to death. This means that individuals who practice fasting can live longer and healthier lives compared to those who don't. Intermittent fasting stimulates the body to repair worn tissue parts, and it has anti-aging benefits. This means that every cell will be kept working as effectively as possible.

5. Understanding hunger

One should learn to decipher body signals accurately, and intermittent fasting is one of the ways for one to understand the hunger cycle. Before the body gets to the real hunger, if it is not fed, it will enter into starvation mode, and you will feel the pangs of hunger that we may attribute to physiological cravings. Such an emotional desire is confused with hunger, but with fasting, practitioners will only experience the real hunger pain in their stomach. One may also experience the detox and withdrawal symptoms that we associate with the consumption of processed foods. With intermittent fasting, one develops a great appreciation for food if you eat after some period of hunger.

6. Stimulating brain function

   Research done about intermittent fasting has found that it has numerous benefits to the health of the brain. Fasting is known to stimulate the brain in a number of different ways. It helps in recovery from strokes, promotes the growth of nerves, and enhances the performance of memory.

Individuals who practice fasting have reduced risks of suffering from neurodegenerative diseases such as Parkinson's or Alzheimer's, and research has shown that intermittent fasting will improve the quality of life and cognitive function of individuals living with that condition.

7. Improved immune system

    Research has shown that intermittent fasting triggers the generation of white blood cells, which are responsible for the immunity of your body. If you fast on short and frequent cycles, the body will be triggered to repair the worn out and damaged immune system cells, and even generate new ones, making your body more secure from attack by diseases. Studies have shown that a 72-hour fast is enough to protect the patients from the toxic and harmful effects that result from chemotherapy treatments. These effects are known to destroy the immune system of the patient. Fasting is also a good way for improving the immune system of elderly individuals.

8. Skin rejuvenation

Individuals with acne are sure that one of the
ways to cure this is through diet, by limiting
the consumption of dairy foods and avoiding
eating processed foods. This means that with
intermittent fasting, one can cure many skin
condition including acne. Most skin conditions
are as a result of food sensitivities, with the
resulting condition being acne and
inflammatory conditions. After going through
fasting, introduce foods one by one, noting any
changes to your skin, and you will be able to
tell the foods that you need to avoid.
Intermittent fasting has been found to be good
for the nails and hair, helping them grow
strong and healthy. Besides feeling good after
starting intermittent fasting, you will also have
a healthy look.

9. Improved spiritual well-being
    This is the reason why most religions practice
    fasting. A lifestyle with fasting included may
    result into a deeper sense of spirituality.
    Practitioners have said that they feel more
    peaceful when fasting, and fasting is good in
    mood regulation through reduction of the
    levels of anxiety and stress. Fasting is normally

recommended as a way of naturally treating a number of sexual and emotional problems. Fasting will make you feel more connected to the world surrounding you, whether you are doing it for spiritual reasons or not, which will give you a positive outlook and clear mind.

10. Lowering oxidative stress

The cause of oxidative stress is the imbalance in the body's release of the reactive oxygen and its related antioxidative defenses. This may lead to cancer and chronic diseases. Unstable molecules, referred to as free radicals, may react with important molecules such as protein and DNA.

Intermittent fasting is known to cause weight loss, and this may lead to reduced levels of oxidative stress, which will prevent the development of unpleasant conditions. Intermittent fasting is also known to lead to a great antioxidant capability, and this should not be overlooked by anyone who is in need of having an improved well-being of their body.

11. Improved heart function

Fasting leads to reduced levels of fat in the body. This has a number of benefits to the

body and especially the cardiac function.
Research has shown that the Mormon
community has a low cardiac mortality, which
can be attributed to the fact that they don't
drink, smoke, or eat meat in large amounts.
The Mormons also practice intermittent
fasting.

Intermittent fasting is a good way of reducing
the cholesterol levels in the body, most
probably the triglycerides, which the body uses
as sources of energy. Less body fat mean that
there is less strain on the kidneys, increasing
the rate of production of growth hormones and
lowering blood pressure. When these are
combined, they will lead to improved function
of the heart.

12. Prevention of cancer

Intermittent fasting promotes the release of
the growth hormone, which is good in reducing
the risk of the individual from suffering from
some types of cancer. With regular eating, the
body is stimulated to produce more and more
new cells, and this can trigger the development
of certain cancer cells. With fasting, the body
will be given rest from this type of activity,

preventing the chances of the new cells becoming cancerous.

Research has also shown that when intermittent fasting is combined with chemotherapy, it will help in tearing down the protection that hinders the immune system from attacking skin cancer and breast cancer cells.

13. Fastens healing and recovery

When one combines fasting with exercise, they can enjoy a number of health benefits. The benefits are even more when the workout is done at the end of the fasting window. Research has shown that after overnight fasting for three weeks, individuals will have a faster post-workout recovery without showing a decrease in performance. Fasting also increases some of the physiological indicators of the body responsible for muscle growth. Healing improves the recovery process and improves one's sleep, and these eating habits will help the body to easily recover from workouts regardless of how intense they may be.

14. Triggers autophagy

During fasting, the body cells undergo the process of autophagy. With time, damaged or dysfunctional proteins builds up within cells, and the autophagy process helps in the removal of this waste material. This process is very important in the repair and detoxification of the body, and increased autophagy has been found to be good in protecting one from a number of diseases such as Alzheimer's and cancer.

Autophagy will help the cells overcome stresses that come from external sources such as lack of important nutrients and internal issues such as pathogens and other disease causing organisms.

Chapter 8- Fasting for Weight Loss

People have used fasting as a tool for weight loss and improved general health. In one of the studies done about intermittent fasting, it was found to be good in fighting obesity just like continuous calorie restriction. It is known to facilitate fat loss while maintaining lean muscle mass.

When eating a ketogenic diet, fasting will force your body into the process of ketosis, a metabolic state for fat burning and weight loss. Individuals who stay in that state for longer get better results. Relying on a ketogenic diet while fasting will help you stay in ketosis, even after stopping the fasting.

Many plans for weight loss involve hours of prep and planning for regular snacks and meals. Planning is a good idea, especially when healthy meals are concerned, but fasting provides you with a way not to worry about planning. You will have a smaller eating window; hence, there is not much food to be worried about during the day.

Which Intermittent Fasting Method Is Best for Weight Loss?

We can't give a 100 percent correct answer to this question. There are different types of intermittent fasting methods, and the best method varies from individual to individual. If you are just beginning fasting for weight loss, you are encouraged to start smaller then improve on a gradual basis as your body adapts to not eating much frequently. That way, the transition will not overwhelm you.

Intermittent fasting is safer and better for weight loss compared to a juice fast, water fast, or any other fad diet. You can begin simple by skipping a meal each day and notice the hunger feelings are not as scary as most people think. You can then advance to better plan like 5:2. Try different methods to find the one that works for you.

Getting Started

The following tips will help you get started with fasting for weight loss:

1. Focus on consistency.

Begin by choosing a single fasting plan, and stick to it to check whether it works out for you. The body is not always comfortable with changes, and it takes some time for it to adjust. Just stick to the plan, and you will enjoy the benefits.

2. Focus on quality.

   It is true that you will be eating less with fasting, but the kind of food you eat is very important for you to lose weight.

3. Stay hydrated.

   When fasting, don't forget to drink water as it is the only thing you will be consuming during the fasting window.

4. Check the level of ketosis.

   If you are fasting to maintain ketosis, then regularly check the levels of ketones. You may feel that your body is in ketosis, but you may be wrong.

Regardless of the fasting method you choose, always focus on nutrient-dense, healthy, and high-fat foods when not fasting so that you may keep on getting optimal nutrition. Fasting will reset your body, and preparing it for clean foods for fat burning will not have any negative impact on the positive results you get from fasting.

When fasting for weight loss, a healthy mindset is of great essence. Fat and weight loss as a result of low calorie intake will only yield positive results if one doesn't overcompensate during the non-fasting times.

Overall, intermittent fasting can be said to be a good tool for weight loss and provides a great alternative to traditional dieting methods such as portion control and calorie counting. Just find what works for you, and stick to it. Focus on taking healthy foods in between the fasts, and the results will be good.

Chapter 9- Fasting and Muscle Gain

Most studies done about intermittent fasting are usually concerned with weight loss. Note that if a weight loss program is followed without exercise, then it will lead to the loss of both fat mass and lean mass. Lean mass refers to every thing other than fat, including muscle. This applies to weight loss achieved through intermittent fasting and other forms of diets. Some studies have found that some amounts of lean mass, about one kg or two pounds, may be lost as a result of intermittent fasting. However, this will take a number of months to become true. This means that muscle loss can only occur if one fasts for a longer period of time but not with the usual fasting periods.

Intermittent fasting can be seen as a good way of losing body fat while maintaining lean mass. After waking up, that is the best time for one to accelerate fat burning. The level of the growth hormone rises, and the body will be turned into a fat burning machine, while at the same time preserving the body's muscle.

While doing intermittent fasting, you don't have to be worried about loss of muscle mass. For one to loose muscle mass, they have to fast for a very long time, for about 72-plus hours. When you do short fasts, you will enjoy all the benefits of fasting while preserving muscle mass. This means that you will avoid all the negative effects associated with long fasts.

When time for eating big comes, especially after an exercise, the sensitivity of insulin will be high, coupled with an increase in nutrient partitioning. With such an environment, the nutrients will be shuttled into the muscles, giving the muscles an opportunity for growth.

It is recommended that individuals should combine muscle building with intermittent fasting. This is because intermittent fasting and muscle building usually go together. In most cases, the loss or gain of muscles is a function of exercise. Eating alone is not enough for one to gain muscle. The only way to muscle gain is exercise, so if you bare worried of losing your muscle during intermittent fasting, exercise. During fasting, hormonal changes occur in the body to give us more energy (from increased adrenaline), keep energy and glucose stores high (burning ketone bodies and fatty acids) and keeps bones and lean muscles.

Dietary Supplements for Muscle Building

If you want to maintain your muscle mass during intermittent fasting, there are dietary supplements that can help you achieve this. However, it will be good for you to consider what time you take the supplements so that the results of fasting are not interfered with.

The most common supplements you can consider for this are creatine and protein.

If you are sure that you get enough protein from your food, there is no need to take protein supplements. However, if you don't, just go ahead and take the supplements. The protein supplements will help a lot if you know you are very active as they will help you improve your exercise performance and muscle size.

Other than the protein supplements, creatine supplements will help in muscle building during fasting. Creatine refers to a molecule naturally found in the body. If you need to increase the level of creatine in your body, just take dietary supplements. The creatine supplements will prove helpful to you especially if you do frequent exercises. Research has shown that creatine increases the strength gain by 5 to 10 percent from weight training. This is a good percentage.

You may be asking yourself, "Should I take creatine, protein, and other supplements during fasting?" The reason you might be asking is that you think they will negatively affect your muscles. As was stated earlier, short term fasts should not raise a concern about muscle loss. More so, some health benefits associated with intermittent fasting are due to the fact that your body doesn't get nutrients. Such stress on your body will prepare it to fight off serious threats like diseases in the future.

After taking supplements with amino acids during fasting, you are sending a signal to your body that you are not fasting. Also, after consuming enough protein during the feeding window, fasting for up to 16 hours will not be detrimental to your body muscles compared to a normal diet.

To conclude, if you want to maintain your muscles during intermittent fasting, combine it with exercise. Always aim to achieve a slow rate of weight loss, and eating enough protein will help you ensure you maintain your body muscles while doing intermittent fasting.

Chapter 10- Fasting for Women

Intermittent fasting has become so popular due to the benefits associated with it. It is true that there are numerous health benefits associated with intermittent fasting, but it may not suit everyone, especially based on the gender of an individual.

Short term fasts have been found to be very good for the health of human beings, but long term fasts may not be good for women due to hormonal imbalance. Some of the effects of long term intermittent fasts in women include early menopause and reproductive issues. It may also make any pre-existing health conditions worse.

Women may enjoy the health benefits associated with intermittent fasting including increased lean muscle mass, sustainable weight loss, more energy, increased response to cell stress, increase sensitivity to insulin, an increase in production of growth hormone, and many others.

Despite all the above benefits, women are naturally more sensitive to starvation signs, making intermittent fasting a bit tricky for women. Once the female body realizes that it is headed to famine, it will increase the release of ghrelin and leptin, which are hunger hormones. These hormones will send a signal to the body that you are hungry and in need of food. If there isn't food for you to survive on, the body will end up shutting down the system responsible for creating another human. That is how the body naturally protects itself from pregnancy, even in cases when you are not pregnant or you are not trying to conceive.

The fact is that the famine is intentionally imposed onto the body, but the body doesn't know this. The body can't tell the difference between intermittent fasting and true fasting, and that is why it will default into using this protective mechanism. The hormonal imbalance brought about by intermittent fasting in women may lead to the following:

- Amenorrhea and irregular periods
- Shrinking of ovaries
- Metabolic stress
- Difficulty sleeping
- Fertility issues
- Anxiety and depression

All the hormones in the female body are highly interconnected, and if any of them is thrown off balance, the rest of the hormones will be affected negatively. This is similar to a domino effect. They are responsible for regulating every function of the body, including digestion, energy production, blood, and metabolism; hence, you should not interrupt their rhythm.

The question now is: Should women practice intermittent fasting? The answer is yes for those who can follow a more relaxed approach. As a female, you can practice intermittent fasting for a brief timeframe, and you will achieve your weight loss goals and achieve the other health goals that we mentioned earlier, and you will not mess up your hormones.

The Best Method

The question is: How can women do intermittent fasting? The following guidelines should director women who want to practice intermittent fasting:

- Avoid fasting for more than 24 hours per session

- Keep your fasts to between 12 to 16 hours
- Avoid fasting on consecutive days during the first two to three weeks of fasting. If, for example, you go for a 16-hour fast, do it for 3 days each week rather than for 7 days. The reason is that the body is yet to adopt to going for such a long period without food.
- Drink a lot of fluids when fasting, for example, herbal tea, bone broth, and water.
- Only do easy exercises when fasting, for examples, yoga, jogging, walking, and stretching.

When Should Women Avoid Intermittent Fasting?

Women should avoid fasting under the following circumstances:

- When nursing
- During pregnancy
- When having difficulty getting to sleep or if you have a sleep disorder
- Have previously had an eating disorder, for example, anorexia and bulimia

- When under chronic stress

Note that intermittent fasting is a way of complementing a healthy lifestyle and diet, but it should not be used as a way of remedying five days of eating foods that are nutritionally-bankrupt like processed foods, refined sugar, and fast foods.

When to Stop

The reproductive system of females is highly intertwined to metabolism. In case you miss periods, just know that your hormones have been disrupted, and not just the ones responsible for getting you pregnant. Naturally, women usually eat less protein compared to men. This will become even less when fasting.

Consumption of less protein means that one is taking in fewer amino acids. Amino acids are essential for activation of estrogen receptors and for synthesis of IGF-1 (insulin-like growth factor) in the liver. The IGF-1 causes the uterine lining to thicken. Diets low in proteins can reduce fertility in women.

Note that the estrogen hormone is not for reproduction only. The estrogen receptors are everywhere in the body, even the brain, bones, and GI tract. A change in estrogen balance will lead to a change in metabolic function, digestion, moods, cognition, bone formation, protein turnover, etc.

For the case of energy balance and appetite, estrogen works in a number of ways. In the brainstem, estrogen is responsible for triggering the peptides that signals you to feel full. If you do anything that causes estrogen to drop, you will end up feeling hungrier.

Women should begin gently with intermittent fasting, and check on their progress regularly. The following are circumstances under which women should stop intermittent fasting:

- Menstrual cycle becomes irregular or stops
- You have sleep problems, either difficult of staying asleep or getting to sleep
- Your hair falls out
- The skin becomes dry or you develop acne
- If it becomes hard to recover from workouts
- If your injuries are taking long to recover from

- If you notice a reduce tolerance to stress.
- If your moods start swinging frequently
- Your heart begins to beat in a weird way
- You notice a reduced interest in romance
- You notice a significant drop in digestion
- When you realize that you are feeling cold most of the time

Notice the category of women we discussed earlier that should not even attempt to fast. Expectant mothers need more energy. If you are planning to start a family, we don't recommend that you fast. If you don't sleep well or are under chronic stress, your body needs to be nurtured but not additionally stressed. If you have experienced an eating disordered in the past, fasting could create more problems for you, so avoid it completely.

You don't have to mess with your health because of fasting. There are several other ways through which you can achieve the health goals you have. If you are just beginning fasting and exercise, then it may be hard for you. Before you can begin fasting, you should first address any nutritional deficiencies that you may have. This will ensure that you first have a solid nutritional foundation. This way, fasting will not bring health problems to you.

If fasting is not for you, and you need to lose weight and achieve other weight goals, consider doing something to the diet you eat.

Crescendo Intermittent Fasting

Whenever you find yourself experiencing the bad symptoms brought about by intermittent fasting, you should stop immediately. It will take a few weeks for the symptoms to stabilize, after which you can try a gentle intermittent fasting. The 5:2 diet is an example of a gentle intermittent fasting.

The question is: How can women fast without experiencing an hormonal imbalance? It is recommended that women should fast on nonconsecutive days. We can call it a crescendo intermittent fasting; one is simply working out the body to find what is suitable for it.

We recommend that you begin with a 12 to 16 hours fast for two days a week, but the days should not be consecutive. During the restricted window, you should only focused on eating healthy foods. For example, from 10:00 AM to 6:00 PM. You can achieve this by not eating breakfast. During the fast days, we recommend that you do some training. However, make it very short, and don't do heavy exercises. We recommend that you do light exercise like HIIT or yoga.

The following are the details of a crescendo intermittent fasting:

1. Fast for two or three nonconsecutive days each week.
2. Do light exercise during fasting days. Examples include strength, yoga, and light studio.
3. Fast for between 12 to 16 hours.
4. During the high-cardio days, eat your meals normally. The high-cardio days include many hours of running, biking, etc.
5. Ensure that you drink plenty of water. You may also drink tea or coffee, but avoid overloading with calories.

By the end of two to three weeks, you will be used to fasting. It is after this that you should fast for longer and add nuances such as fasting for longer during the weekends and holidays and fasting shorter during the weekdays.

Part 3

Nutrition

Chapter 11- The Most Common Intermittent Fasting Mistakes

Intermittent fasting is associated with a number of benefits including an improved general well-being. It only involves limiting the number of hours that you eat in a day. Most people use intermittent fasting as a complement for a low carb diet, paleo diet, or ketogenic diet. Intermittent fasting can be done in a number of ways, but in all of these, it only involves not eating what you used to eat for 12 to 18 hours. The good thing with this is that it mostly happens during the night, making it easy for people to get through.

Despite the many advantages of intermittent fasting, some people struggle or fail to see the benefits for their health. Others find it easy to follow the intermittent fasting lifestyle in terms of the eating schedule. The main cause of this must be that there is something they are doing wrong. This means the method or approach you follow toward intermittent fasting will mark your success or failure.

Fasting should improve your general health. However, if it makes you feel moody, sluggish, or too hungry, there is a possibility that you are making any of the following mistakes:

Failure to eat enough healthy foods

When one is intermittent fasting, they are expected to nourish their bodies with whole and nutrient-dense foods. People think that intermittent fasting works like magic by solving all their problems, but this will not occur if you don't eat healthy foods. In a fasting state, the body begins to break down the damaged components then uses them as sources of energy, a process responsible for cleaning and healing the body. Another effect of this is that the body will become more sensitive to the food you eat, and it will be good for this to be nutrient-dense food. However, it will not be good if you are not eating healthy foods. If you don't nourish your body with foods that are dense in nutrients, it will mean that you will feel hungry all the time as the body will crave certain nutrients.

After the fasting window is over, most people rush to eat so as to feel full. Here, one can easily make the mistake of eating food that doesn't provide them with all the nutrients they need, making them feel full. This means that they don't have room to eat other foods that should provide them with these nutrients. This is a poor eating habit during fasting. It is recommended during the eating window, one should get high-fat, nutrient-dense foods and make them part of their diet. This way, you will be able to get the calories that your body needs and enough nutrients as you need. This way, you will be able to meet your caloric needs.

Adding creamers

Most creamers are rich in calories. Coffee is good during fasting, but when you add creamers to it, it is no longer good. The reason is that when you add creamers to the coffee, it is no longer a drink but a food. This will break your fasting. Creamers will trigger a metabolic response when consumed. The goal of intermittent fasting is to make the body burn the stored fats in the form of glycogen for energy. If you take coffee with creamers, the body will try to burn the calories provided by the creamers; hence, it will break from burning the stored fats, meaning that you are no longer fasting. If you need to drink coffee during fasting, avoid adding creamers to it however small the amount. Otherwise, you may not see the benefits of intermittent fasting.

Eating branched-chain amino acids

Branched-chain amino acids are known to break a fast. The reason is that branched-chain amino acids cause a rise in the levels of insulin in the body. The overall effect of this is a stop of the detoxification process. The body will also stop burning stored fats for energy. Some people may argue that branched-chain amino acids only cause a small spike in insulin. However, note that any time the insulin level goes up during fasting, it is similar to starting the fasting process afresh. Branched-chain amino acids should be avoided during intermittent fasting.

Not drinking enough water

One should stay hydrated during intermittent fasting. Intermittent fasting is known to trigger the process of cell apoptosis. This process simply involves cell death and recycling. The process involves killing all the damaged cells and the ones that are not needed. These should be secreted or removed from the body. If you don't take enough water, then these toxins will not be secreted. This means that the body will kill the unwanted cells but will not able to remove them.

Also, during intermittent fasting, one breaks up a lot of fat that has been stored in the body. There are a lot of toxins that are stored in body fat. If you don't drink enough water during fasting, the body will break down the fats but fail to secrete the toxins. This means that the toxins will still stay in the body. This will make the body cells toxic. When fasting, ensure that you take a lot of water.

Not taking your minerals

Minerals like potassium, magnesium, and others are so critical when one is fasting. The minerals will not affect your calorie intake. Minerals are very essential, especially when one is drinking a lot of water during fasting. Minerals play a significant role in the cellular functions of the body and the function of the brain in sending electrical signals throughout the body. If the body doesn't have adequate minerals, then these won't function well.

You must ensure that you get a lot of sodium during fasting. You can add ¼ or ½ teaspoon of this to your water. This will make the walls of the body cells more permeable, meaning that they will allow toxins to move in and out. This will mean that you stay hydrated during the fasting period, and you give the body the ability to secrete toxins.

Fasting for many days in a week

When doing intermittent fasting, most people believe that the more days they do it, the better. Overtraining may lead to a lack of sleep or injury, and in the same way, overdoing intermittent fasting may result in counterproductive effects.

It is recommended that one should fast for two to four days each week. Fasting for more than this may affect performance, metabolism, and appetite since the body will begin to fight any perceived starvation. Also, one must check the fasting window during intermittent fasting. If the window is too long, it will trigger extreme hunger that may make you binge.

In most cases, it takes some time to know the intermittent fasting method that fits you in terms of the number of days to fast every week and how long the fast should last for each day. It can take trial and error for one to know the method to stick to. When beginning intermittent fasting, we recommend that you start small, maybe one to two fasts per week. Ensure each fast goes for 12 to 24 hours. After you get used to this routine, you can go ahead and add one more day to the routine. Instead of adding a day, you may consider prolonging your fasting period from 12 to 14 hours to maybe 14 to 18 hours. However, always do what you find yourself comfortable doing.

Intense training

It is true that there are some people who will be okay with intense exercise during intermittent fasting, especially when you are already healthy or you are used to being active most of the time. However, for most individuals practicing intermittent fasting, they will feel okay when resting during the fasting period. Others may also need more sleep during intermittent fasting.

Experts have recommended that one should skip intense workouts during intermittent fasting like long aerobic training sessions or HIIT, especially on days when you take in less fuel. Instead of going for long training sessions, it is recommended that you go for gentler, restorative workouts such as yoga or walking outside. These are known to be the best exercises for one during fasting to help them avoid fatigue, weakness, or dizziness.

However, you must always note that having adequate sleep is very essential during fasting. Adequate is good for proper digestion, body repair, detoxification, and balancing of body hormones. Always sleep for 7 to 9 hours each day to avoid low energy, cravings, and moodiness.

Accelerating the fat burning potential of the body

Combining intermittent fasting with a fat burner is a good choice. This means that selecting the right supplement can give you good results after fasting. You must eat the right diet and do the right exercises. The right burner will help you lose the extra body weight on your stomach. A fat burner will help you accelerate the rate of metabolism; hence, you will burn more calories each day. It will also suppress hunger, making you feel less hungry. It will help you stay more energetic throughout the day despite the fact that you are fasting. There will be less water retention.

This means that if you really need to lose fat, it will be good for you to include a fat burner into your fasting. This will give you best results. However, ensure that you choose the best fat burner.

Counting minutes to the eating window

When fasting, some people will keep on staring at the clock for the eating window to come. This is an indication that something is wrong. This is why you should not stay idle during fasting, but be focused on other things like your family, career, friends, and even planning your next vacation. If, for example, you bare fasting for 16 hours, half of this time, that is, 8 hours, should be spent sleeping.

Instead of breaking from what you were doing to go for a meal, intermittent fasting will provide you with time to focus on other things. It is a fasting method designed to make your life easier.

The only thing that should worry you during intermittent fasting is real hunger that normally occurs after 16 to 24 hours, but not after 4 hours. Only the body should dictate to you when to eat, rather than the clock. If you focus more on the clock to eat, then you will be able to learn to listen to your body signals.

Being afraid of getting hungry

During intermittent fasting, one will be getting hungry from time to time. This should be the goal of intermittent fasting. When you get hungry, the body turns to burning stored fat to get energy. The reason is that the body doesn't have carbs to process for energy; hence, the alternative is burning the stored fat. This leads to weight loss.

However, a number of people believe that once they feel hungry, their body will be going catabolic, and they will end up losing muscle. However, the fact remains that it's possible for you to go without eating for long periods of time, even 24 hours in some cases.

This will depend on how you have planned to do your intermittent fasting. You don't have to be afraid of getting hungry. Anytime you feel hungry, just know that you are giving your body an opportunity to burn the stored fat. After some time, you will see the benefits, which will be manifested by well-being including weight loss.

Choosing the wrong plan

Intermittent fasting takes different forms, and that's why you should choose the best one based on your needs, lifestyle and schedule. When choosing a plan, consider the demands of your job, family, and workout program.

Giving up too quickly

Intermittent fasting requires one to be disciplined, and it will take some time for one to get used to it. One will find it tough during the first four to five days. One will feel hungry, lightheaded, get headaches, or feel exhausted. You should note that the feelings will pass quickly, and before the end of the first week, your body will be used to intermittent fasting. The hunger will disappear, and you will begin to feel more energetic and focused.

In case you don't begin to feel better by the end of the first week, there might be something wrong, most probably overdoing it when it is too early. You may also have chosen the wrong plan. Most people give up on intermittent fasting immediately after trying. The reason is that they fear getting hungry. Before beginning intermittent fasting, you must know that the first few days will be challenging to you, so be ready for this.

Eating too little

Fasting will affect the hormones responsible for appetite in your body, and you may end up not feeling hungry after you get used to intermittent fasting. During the eating window, you may find yourself eating only a small portion. However, it will be good for you to ensure that you don't take in too few calories. Failure to eat enough may make you feel so hungry the following day, which may prevent you from performing your work. This can force you not to fast that day. This means that eating too little during the eating window is not good.

Chapter 12- Intermittent Fasting Fluids

The best fluids for intermittent fasting are the ones with no calories or those that are low in calories. There are various drinks one can consume during intermittent fasting, but the key is, ensure there are no calories. Let us explore the fluids that one can take during intermittent fasting.

Tea and Coffee

Tea is recommended as a drink for intermittent fasting since it has less calories that cannot frustrate your weight loss efforts. The tea should be taken plain without milk, cream, or sugar. You can drink either hot or cold tea, and all will be well. Some artificial sweeteners are allowed for those in need of sweetening their tea.

Coffee can be consumed during intermittent fasting, but ensure you drink only black coffee. The coffee should also be taken without milk, sugar, or cream as they have calories. Artificial sweeteners can help you add flavor to the coffee. Coffee drinks sold in coffee shops should be avoided as most of them have milk products, syrup, or sugary add-ins.

Water

Fasting is good and healthy, but if water is avoided for longer periods of time, it can turn out to be dangerous. The body is in need of water to stay hydrated, and lack of this for longer durations may lead to health problems. Examples of such health problems include brain swelling, seizures, kidney failure, heat stroke, and even death. It is recommended that you add maple syrup and lemon juice to the water for additional flavor and energy. You may also add some vegetables into the water, boil them, remove them, then drink what you are left with. Such a drink will have some nutrients that will add some flavor to the water that you drink.

Juice

Juice cannot be said to be free of calories. This makes it not good for short fasts. However, individuals doing longer fasts are in need of some energy and strength to carry them through that period. Juice is the best source of nutrients for this. Ensure that you only drink juice that is 100 percent vegetable or fruit since they are the best in terms of nutrition. They are rich in vitamins A, C, iron, and potassium. These are good sources of energy to enable you to go through the fasting period. Other than that, you will at least have something to put into your mouth which will in turn motivate you to get through the fast.

Baking Soda

Most people use baking soda for cooking purposes only, but it has numerous health benefits. It relieves us from bloat and constipation. It aids the process of digestion. Baking soda will neutralize all the acidity in your gut while killing bacteria and parasites. After consuming baking soda, you will have balanced the PH levels in your body.

A teaspoon of baking soda in your water will help you boost health and physical performance during fasting. Fasting works to remove minerals and water; hence, it will be good for you to regularly check on the level of electrolytes in your body.

Baking soda is made up of 100 percent sodium bicarbonate which can provide you with sodium when fasting. It has a bad taste that will help you prevent hunger during fasting. Once you have taken baking soda, you will not want to eat anything, and this will help you continue with the fast.

Herbal Teas

Herbal teas have a great taste which can help one fight off hunger during fasting. They are also good at detoxifying the body as well as other medicinal benefits.

A cup of herbal tea has only one to five calories, which cannot interrupt your efforts to lose weight. However, avoid brewing tea with berries, fruits, or any other type with carbohydrates. The sugar in such teas will frustrate your weight loss efforts.

Apple Cider Vinegar

Apple cider vinegar has anti-inflammatory and antibacterial compounds that make it good for fasting. Its acidic nature will help you balance the levels of PH in your body. Apple cider vinegar has no calories, but it has other nutrients like potassium, iron, and some magnesium. These are very good for fasting individuals as it will help them check on their electrolytes and prevent any deficiencies that may occur.

The apple cider vinegar will also kill bad bacteria from your gut and prevent hunger. Add it to sparkling water, and you will end up with a tasty beverage. To keep the process autophagy going, we recommend you add one to two tablespoons of apple cider vinegar each time. Apple cider vinegar can be consumed during fasts, but it is a great way of breaking from fasts. In such a case, some squeezed lemon juice should be added to create digestive enzymes, and the gut will be prepared for eating.

Artificial Sweeteners

Artificial sweeteners can be used during fasting, but the kind of sweetener you take is of great importance. Bodies react differently to different artificial sweeteners.

Artificial sweeteners like dextrose, maltodextrin, or sucralose have carbohydrates in them; hence, they should be avoided completely. A natural sweetener like stevia has not shown any sign of raising blood sugar or insulin, making it good for drinking during intermittent fasting. However, ensure that you are aware of how your body reacts to stevia. Stevia has no calories in it, but it is 300 times sweeter compared to table sugar; hence, it can result in placebo-like insulin response. This will stimulate your taste buds, and your body will no longer be in a fasting state.

Glauber's Salts

If you are doing intermittent fasting for improved health and for cellular cleansing, Glauber's salt will be good for you. Glauber's salt is used in medicine for triggering bowel movements. Once 5 to 20 grams of

Glauber's salt are added to water, one can do away with constipation, clean the digestive tract, and reduce bloat. However, avoid over-consuming this as it can lead to diarrhea and dehydration.

If you take in only the drinks above, then you will see good results from intermittent fasting.

Chapter 13- Foods to Eat

Intermittent fasting is taking the world by storm. The reason might be that there are no strict food rules. You are restricted on when to eat, but not what to eat. In intermittent fasting, there are no much restrictions on the type of food to eat and the amount to eat. A balanced diet is essential for weight loss, sticking to a diet, and maintaining energy levels. Individuals in need of losing weight should eat foods rich in nutrients. Examples of such foods include fruits, veggies, nuts, beans, whole grains, seeds, lean proteins, and dairy products. The best foods are the ones recommended for improved health, high in fiber, whole foods, and unprocessed foods.

Let us discuss the foods that should be eaten during intermittent fasting:

Avocado

It may sound funny to eat this high-calorie fruit during fasting. However, avocado is rich in monounsaturated fat which is very satiating. A study has found that adding half of an avocado to your lunch will keep you full for longer compared to eating the lunch without avocado. Make this fruit part of your diet when doing intermittent fasting.

Fish

Most dietary guidelines propose eating no less than eight ounces of fish every week. The fish is rich in proteins and healthy fats, and it provides plenty of vitamin D to the body. This is the right food to eat during fasting as it will provide your body with many nutrients at one time. Since you are consuming a low number of calories during intermittent fasting, this may affect your cognition, but fish will improve this since it is termed as "brain food."

Cruciferous Veggies

Veggies like cauliflower, brussels sprouts, and broccoli are rich in fiber. When fasting, fiber is of great importance in helping you prevent constipation and keep you regular. Fiber is also capable of making you feel full, and this is good, especially if you are going to go for 16 hours without eating. Ensure the cruciferous veggies are part of your diet during intermittent fasting.

Potatoes

Always remember that not all white foods are bad. Studies have found that potatoes are one of the most satiating foods. Another study has shown that eating potatoes as part of a healthy diet can help in weight loss. Note that potato chips and french fries don't count.

Beans and Legumes

Anything added to chili should be good for intermittent fasting. Carbs provide the body with energy for activity. Avoid overloading carbs, but it is recommendable that you add in some low-calorie carbs to your diet during intermittent fasting. Beans and legumes are good for this. Foods such as chickpeas, peas, black beans, and lentils have been found to be good for reducing weight even without restricting intake for calories.

Probiotics

The critters in your gut like diversity and consistency. These will never be happy anytime you feel hungry. Any time your gut is not happy, you may experience a number of problems including constipation. This can be countered by taking probiotic-rich foods such as kraut, kombucha, or kefir. Gut shots will be good for any day you need to take 500 calories since every 1.5 ounce shot has live probiotics for only 10 calories.

Berries

Berries are good for making a smoothie full of nutrients. Berries are a good source of vitamin C which is good for boosting the immune system. A cup of berries will provide you with over 100 percent of the daily value of vitamin C. Berries such as strawberries and blueberries are rich in flavonoids. Individuals who consume flavonoids usually have a smaller BMI compared to those who don't. This is another importance of eating berries.

Eggs

Eggs can be cooked up within minutes, and one egg contains six grams of protein. Eating protein will help you build muscle and stay full during intermittent fasting. Research has found that men who eat an egg for breakfast, rather than a bagel, felt fuller and ate less during the whole day. If you are doing intermittent fasting, and you need to increase your fast window, then hard-boil some eggs and eat them. This will reduce the pangs of hunger; hence, you will fast for a longer period.

Nuts

Nuts may have many calories compared to other snacks, but they have one advantage; they are rich in good fats. Research has shown that the polyunsaturated fats contained in walnuts can change the physiological markers for satiety and hunger.

You also don't have to be worried about calories when eating nuts. A study done in 2012 found that a one-ounce serving of almonds (which is about 23 nuts) has 20 percent less calories than what is listed on the label. When chewing, the walls of the almond cells will not be broken down completely; hence, a portion of the nuts you eat will be left intact, and they won't be absorbed during digestion. This means that nuts will not give you as many calories as one might think.

Whole Grains

Eating carbs while fasting may seem to be strange, but this is not the case all the time. Whole grains are rich in proteins and fiber; hence, eating some during fasting will help you stay full longer. Research has also shown that consumption of whole grains, rather than refined grains, may increase the rate of metabolism in the body. This is why you should not leave out whole grains when fasting. Some of the best whole grains include farro, bulgur, kamut, amaranth, spelt, sorghum, millet, and freekeh.

Chapter 14- Intermittent Fasting and Keto Diet

The keto diet is a low-carb, high-fat diet good for weight loss. It is also good for improved body energy and regulated blood sugar. The goal of intermittent fasting is to cut down one's eating window to aid in weight loss and other benefits.

Both of these two diets are great for body health. Can the two work together?

With fasting, one can be left feeling very hungery, especially before they get used to the new eating pattern. The good thing with the keto diet is that it can reduce cravings and hunger. With the keto diet, one can go for a long time without eating food. This means that intermittent fasting and the keto diet can work together successfully.

With intermittent fasting, the levels of ketones can be kept at a high level by keeping a low level of insulin hormone. This way, one can reduce their appetite and burn fat for fuel. It is true that these two diets have nearly the same health benefits to the body; hence, they work together for improved results.

How to Do it

Ketosis and intermittent fasting should not be short term diets. If the diet is working great for you, there is no need for you to do it for a short time. However, before continuing, ensure that your doctor confirms your health is good, and you are not starving all the time.

If any eating pattern seems appealing to you, you don't have to worry about trying it. However, ensure that you first talk to a qualified and trusted health professional regarding your condition to tell you whether it is safe for you or not. During intermittent fasting and the keto diet, always ensure you consume bulletproof coffee and avocadoes.

If you need to know the fasting window that is best for you, just pay attention to how you feel. Always check your hunger levels, energy levels, sleep quality, and cognitive function.

If you find that you are finding it hard to maintain that fasting window, or you can't go for a workout, then you need to reduce your fasting window. This can then be increased by one hour for every week.

You can also choose to reduce the number of days that you fast. During the feeding window, ensure that you take in adequate calories. Work closely with a nutritionist or dietician to determine the number of calories you need on a daily basis based on the level of your activity, unique body composition, and lifestyle factors.

Intermittent fasting can be imposed on a keto diet just like any other diet, such as Paleo, as the same rules will apply. The main advantage of imposing intermittent fasting on a keto diet is that it will trigger the process of ketosis faster, helping you reach your health goals sooner.

The following simple schedules can help you get started with intermittent fasting on a keto diet:

1. Eat between 9:00 AM-9:00 PM, fast for 12 hours.
2. Eat between 9:00 AM-7:00 PM, fast for 14 hours.
3. Eat between 12:00-8:00 PM, fast for 16 hours (16/8 method).

Who Should Not Fast on the Keto Diet?

The keto diet during intermittent fasting may be good for most people, but it is not recommended for everyone. If you know you have had some hormonal conditions, this is not for you. If your gallbladder has been removed, then avoid both keto diet and intermittent fasting. Individuals suffering from diabetes, hypoglycemia (low blood sugar), kidney disease, and those who have had an eating disorders should avoid it as it could trigger symptoms. If you are nursing or expectant, do not fast on a keto diet. Individuals with sleeping disorders should also not fast.

Benefits of Intermittent Fasting on the Keto Diet

The following are the benefits you will enjoy after imposing intermittent fasting on a keto diet:

1. Getting into ketosis sooner
   The keto diet denies the body of its fuel which are carbs. Combining this with intermittent fasting will send the body into ketosis sooner.

The keto diet briefly introduces you into fasting; hence, it will be easy for you to fast for longer durations of time. Some researchers have stated that fasting on a keto diet will help you reduce the symptoms of keto flu.

2. Improved rate of weight loss
The keto diet works in different ways to break the weight loss plateaus. First, a keto diet helps the body break down stored fat for energy rather than breaking down carbs, meaning the process of metabolism is stimulated to burn fats faster. Fat usually takes a longer period of time to break down, meaning that they will make you feel full for longer. This way, you will avoid snacking and intake of calories during the fasting window.
When intermittent fasting is combined with the keto diet, the eating window will be made smaller, and any food you eat will be used by the body as the fuel, and you won't feel deprived or hungry.

3. Regulating blood sugar
Intermittent fasting and the keto diet have been found to be good in improving insulin sensitivity which is stabilizes blood sugar

levels. This is good for weight loss. Since these two are good for one to achieve stable blood sugar level, when combined, they will be helpful to individuals suffering from type-2 diabetes. With a stable blood sugar, one will eliminate brain fog, improve concentration, focus, and memory.

4. Improved nutrient absorption

    Research has shown that the absorption of protein and carbs is more efficient after doing a workout before a meal. This is an indication that fasting will make the body use the nutrients from the previous post-workout meals in a more efficient manner. This will lead to accelerated growth of lean muscle mass and an improvement in your general health.

5. Natural detoxification

    The keto diet and intermittent fasting are capable of triggering the process of autophagy which was discussed previously. This is the process through which worn out cell parts are repaired so that the body may have healthy cells.

    Autophagy takes place naturally during fasting, or during periods when your intake of carbs and protein is low. When intermittent fasting and a keto diet are combined, this process will be accelerated. This is good for your health as you will have a reduced risk of type 2 diabetes and cardiovascular disease.

It is true that a combination of intermittent fasting and a keto diet can help you reach your health goals faster, but you should always remember that the two diets are designed to be practiced as part of a healthy lifestyle. There are a few things that may be used to replace a diet that is rich in nutrient dense foods.

If you have just started to eat the keto diet, it is advisable that you allow your body to get used to it for three to four weeks before beginning to practice intermittent fasting on the keto diet.

Chapter 15- Sample Meal Plan

For effective weight loss, one must choose what works for them. If you feel like eating breakfast, eat it. If you don't feel like it, don't worry. It is still possible for you to you to lose weight and remain healthy.

If you need to eat six meals each day for body building, go ahead. If it works well for you and for your lifestyle, be grateful. However, that is not the only way to lose weight. One can eat one to two meals per day, and at the same time, lose weight and feel very good.

It was once believed that one must eat at least once every two to three hours to keep their metabolism going. Intermittent fasting may even increase the rate of metabolism while eating at this rate may reduce the rate of metabolism as a result of a reduced insulin sensitivity.

For one to lose weight, one of the goals should be to get all the nutrients needed by the body. This has proven to be hard as some people don't get all the nutrients that are needed for consumption every day.

Nutrient deficiencies should first be addressed before getting into a weight loss journey.

Intermittent fasting imposes social barriers to those practicing it, and this has made it a challenge for people to follow it. Many people are used to holding social events during breakfast, lunch, and dinner. They have learned to eat during breakfast, lunch, and dinner ever since they were born. Eating three meals a day seems to fit the lifestyle of nearly every individual on earth.

Three Meals a Day

The protocol of eating three meals a day, combined with occasional fasting period, is applicable to the life of nearly everyone. The reason is that most people are already used to eating three meals a day during breakfast, lunch, and dinner.

You are allowed to eat meals at the frequency that you need to get all the nutrients into your body. However, you must avoid eating too many calories, stimulating insulin too much and getting frustrated and hungry with missing meals. The three-meal per day eating plan coupled with intermittent fasting can work miracles. The protocol below can be followed:

- The base protocol is that you will be eating three meals each day. Ninety percent of the time you will be eating three meals per day, for about six to seven days every week. This way, you will have a room to miss a meal every day and do a fast after overeating or when you realize you made a poor food choice.

- You can drink one super shake everyday together with two other meals. The time the meals are consumed is not of importance. Your goal should be to ensure you choose nutrient-dense foods and ensure that the portion size is a match with your caloric needs and body type.

- Intermittent fasting should be practiced when you need to. It should be practiced after overeating, 16 to 20 hours before planning to overeat, partake of some not so healthy foods, or in cases you need to travel, and you don't want to eat unhealthy foods.

There are no magic tricks in this, but it is as simple as that! You only have to drink a super shake every day alongside two other meals that correctly match your nutrient needs. A fast can be as simple as pushing the reset button to cleanse the body after eating an unhealthy meal. Note that you should focus on eating three meals most days.

The three-meal per day template can be made based on the time you go for a workout. In this case, I have prepared some templates based on the times you do the workout.

Morning Workout

Pre-workout:

Two scoops of amino-acids (branched-chain) with 250-350 grams of whey protein powder or 17-25 ounces of water. You don't need carbs as you have already stored glycogen good for the morning workout.

Meal One

This should be a super shake. Choose protein, fruit, green food, and fat, and blend it with water and ice.

Meal Two

- 1-2 protein palms. Choose organic chicken, organic eggs, grass-fed beef, etc.

- 0.5-2 handfuls of carbohydrates (cupped). Choose sweet potatoes, quinoa, or jasmine rice.
- 1-2 vegetable fistfuls. Choose broccoli, asparagus, peppers, cruciferous veggies, leafy greens, etc.
- 1-2 thumbs of fat. Choose extra virgin olive oil, avocados, or almonds.

Meal Three

- 1-2 palms of protein. Choose organic chicken, organic eggs, grass-fed beef, etc.
- 0.5-2 handfuls of carbohydrates (cupped). Choose sweet potatoes, quinoa, or jasmine rice.
- 1-2 vegetable fistfuls. Choose broccoli, asparagus, peppers, cruciferous veggies, leafy greens, etc.
- 1-2 thumbs of fat. Choose extra virgin olive oil, avocados, or almonds.

Afternoon Workout

Meal One:

This should be a super shake. Choose protein, fruit, green food, and fat, and blend it with water and ice.

You can also choose:

- 1-2 palms of protein. Choose organic eggs or grass-fed whey protein
- 0.5-2 handfuls of carbohydrates (cupped). Choose steel rolled or cut oats, berries, or any other fruit.
- 1-2 vegetable fistfuls. Choose broccoli, asparagus, peppers, leafy greens, or cruciferous veggies
- 1-2 thumbs of fat. Choose nuts and seeds, grass-fed butter, or extra virgin coconut oil.

Pre-Workout:

Two scoops of amino-acids (branched-chain) with 250-350 grams of whey protein powder or 17-25 ounces of water. For improved gains in muscle mass, add some carbs.

Meal Two:

This should be a super shake. Choose protein, fruit, green food, and fat, and blend it with water and ice.

Meal Three:

- 1-2 palms of protein. Choose organic chicken eggs or grass-fed beef, etc.

- 0.5-2 handfuls of carbohydrates (cupped). Choose sweet potatoes, quinoa, or jasmine rice.

- 1-2 vegetable fistfuls. Choose broccoli, asparagus, peppers, leafy greens, or cruciferous veggies

- 1-2 thumbs of fat. Choose extra virgin olive oil, avocados, or almonds.

Evening/Night Time Workout

Meal One

This should be a super shake. Choose protein, fruit, green food, and fat, and blend it with water and ice.

You can also choose:

- 1-2 palms of protein. Choose organic eggs or grass-fed whey protein

- 0.5-2 handfuls of carbohydrates (cupped). Choose steel rolled or cut oats, berries, or any other fruit.

- 1-2 vegetable fistfuls. Choose broccoli, asparagus, peppers, or leafy greens.

- 1-2 thumbs of fat. Choose nuts and seeds, grass-fed butter, or extra virgin coconut oil.

Meal Two

- 1-2 palms of protein. Choose organic chicken, organic eggs, or grass-fed beef, etc.

- 0.5-2 handfuls of carbohydrates (cupped). Choose sweet potatoes, quinoa, or jasmine rice.

- 1-2 vegetable fistfuls. Choose broccoli, asparagus, peppers, leafy greens, or cruciferous veggies

- 1-2 thumbs of fat. Choose extra virgin olive oil, avocados, almonds, or grass-fed butter.

Pre-Workout

Two scoops of amino-acids (branched-chain) with 250-350 grams of whey protein powder or 17-25 ounces of water.

Meal Three

This should be a super shake. Choose protein, fruit, green food, and fat, and blend it with water and ice.

Those are the templates. The one you choose is up to you. People have different bodies, schedules, and activity levels. This is why you have to find what works for you. Make sure that you get enough sleep, drink adequate water, eat adequate protein, eat a lot of veggies, carbs, and fats, and meal frequency will not matter to you. You must also look for an eating schedule that is good for you, then stick to it.

Conclusion

This marks the end of this guide. Intermittent fasting is associated with a number of benefits. It is concerned more with when you eat rather than what you eat. The individual is provided with the flexibility of eating whatever they need, but they are restricted on the eating period. In most cases, one is required to fast for 12 to 16 hours in a day. During these hours, one is not expected to eat anything that ads calories to the body. However, they are allowed to consume non-caloric drinks such as coffee. One should avoid adding ingredients that will add calories to the coffee. Examples of these are creamers. One then eats during the rest of the hours. During the eating window, one can eat whatever they need. However, one should not binge so that they don't counter the effects of fasting. Intermittent fasting is a good way for one to lose weight naturally. Our bodies need energy for various functions. This energy is obtained from the carbs that we eat. During fasting, we don't eat, meaning that the body doesn't use carbs for energy. In such a case, the body turns to the fats that have been stored in the body. These are burned through the process of metabolism to generate energy that is needed by the body. When these fats are burned, one shows a loss of weight. The fat stored in the body is the major cause of chronic diseases such as diabetes and heart attack. This shows that intermittent fasting is a good way of curing these naturally. It also helps one stay safe from such chronic diseases. Intermittent fasting should be combined with exercise for better results. However, exercise should not be intense but gentle. An example of a gentle exercise is yoga. Women should be careful when practicing intermittent fasting. The reason is that it may lead to hormonal imbalance. Women with special conditions like pregnancy, hormonal imbalance, and other conditions should not try intermittent fasting.

About the Author

James Statton is a nutritionist with several years of experience in the diet and nutrition industry. He also has a strong academic background in this field. He believes that dieting is the best way of curing chronic diseases like diabetes. Proper dieting is key in preventing chronic diseases like cancer and diabetes. He has helped many type-2 diabetic patients to reverse the condition through dieting. James has written several books about preventing chronic diseases through proper dieting. He is a fitness expert with several years of experience practicing yoga.